The Ultimate Guide to Metabolic and Hormonal Health

The Science-Based Method to Boost Metabolism, Balance Hormones, and Burn Fat After 40

AP Elite Health

AP Elite Health

Contents

Introduction

Bridging the Gap - Uniting Mind, Body, and Health with the AP Elite Blueprint

Welcome back to your journey toward lasting health and freedom from the yo-yo dieting cycle that has trapped so many in their pursuit of health and happiness. In our first book, "The Yo-Yo Diet Recovery Handbook: From Fad to Freedom," we debunked tons of diet myths, learned how to overcome emotional hurdles, and improved our own health overall. Together, we navigated beyond the allure of quick fixes and fad diets, laying the foundation for a deeper, more sustainable approach to health—one rooted in understanding and listening to your body.

However, the path to true wellness does not end with breaking free from the cycle of yo-yo dieting. In fact, that's only just the beginning! You deserve a transformation that leaves you not only feeling healed, but better than ever. It's a continual journey of growth, learning, and adaptation.

> **That's where the R4 Transformation System comes into play—a comprehensive, scientifically-backed approach designed by AP Elite Health to take you from merely surviving to thriving.**

This innovative system is our proven blueprint for lasting transformation, guiding you through the essential phases of Rebalance,

Revitalize, Reshape, and Retain. Each phase is a carefully crafted step on the path to not just achieving your health and fitness goals but surpassing them in ways you never imagined possible.

The importance of metabolic health and hormone balance cannot be overstated. These critical components of your overall well-being influence everything from your energy levels and weight to your mood and long-term health. Understanding and optimizing these factors are at the heart of our R4 Transformation System. It's not simply about losing weight; it's about creating a body and life that feel good from the inside out. It's about giving you the tools and knowledge to maintain your transformation, no matter what life throws your way.

As we delve into the R4 Transformation System, remember that this is more than just a method; it's a journey. A journey that requires patience, commitment, and a willingness to embrace change. But you won't be walking this path alone. The principles, strategies, and insights contained in this book, coupled with the support of our community here at AP Elite Health, can be your guideposts.

So, take a deep breath, and let's step forward together. The next chapter of your health and fitness journey begins now, and it's filled with promise, potential, and the power to truly transform. Welcome to *The AP Elite Health Blueprint: Mastering Your Metabolic Health and Body Transformation*. Your adventure to lasting health and ultimate control over your body continues here.

Chapter 1
Understanding the R4 Transformation System

The journey to reclaiming your health, vitality, and control over your body is not a linear path—it unfolds as a dynamic exploration of self-awareness, adaptation, and transformation. The R4 Transformation System encapsulates this expedition, designed around four pivotal phases: Rebalance, Revitalize, Reshape, and Retain. This holistic methodology does not merely offer a program; it's a whole new paradigm for achieving health by addressing the foundational causes of metabolic and hormonal imbalances, steering you toward sustainable change. Let's start by going over the 4 steps of the system so that you know what to expect!

The 4 Steps of the R4 System

1. **Rebalance:** The journey commences with correcting hormonal imbalances and repairing metabolic damage, laying the groundwork for your transformation by restoring your body's natural rhythms. Focused on nutrition, sleep, and stress management, this phase kickstarts the healing process and gets your body not only back to normal, but keeps you feeling amazing throughout the start of your transformation.

2. **Revitalize:** Building on a balanced foundation, we elevate your metabolic health, establishing a metabolic set point. This phase is marked by nutritional strategies and exercise regimens tailored to boost your metabolism, ensuring sustained energy and resilience. This is also where we'll create a routine you'll love and sustain, hence the title, revitalize!

3. **Reshape:** The transformative phase, where body composition and hormonal synergies are refined. Here, the physical transformation becomes visible as we optimize hormonal function to develop lean muscle and shed stubborn fat, revealing a firmer, more toned physique.

4. **Retain:** The culmination of your journey, focusing on solidifying your gains and maintaining your improved health and transformed body for the long term. This phase reinforces sustainable lifestyle changes, equipping you with the tools and habits necessary to maintain your results and continue thriving for the years to come.

The Science Behind the System

At its heart, the R4 Transformation System acknowledges the importance of metabolic health and hormone balance as critical to weight management and overall health. Hormones, the body's chemical messengers, regulate every facet of our health, influencing energy levels, appetite, body composition, and mood.

The journey towards sustainable health and weight management is fraught with challenges, evidenced by the statistics that highlight the struggles many face. It's widely reported that up to 95% of diets fail, with most individuals regaining their lost weight within one to five years. This high failure rate underscores the complexity of weight loss and the need for approaches that go beyond simple calorie restriction.

Studies also suggest that approximately two-thirds of dieters end up heavier than they were before dieting – especially yo-yo dieting. This rebound effect not only discourages further attempts at weight loss but can also lead to a cycle of yo-yo dieting that is detrimental to both physical and mental health.

These statistics highlight the need for a holistic and informed approach, like the R4 Transformation System, which addresses the underlying causes of weight management struggles, including hormonal imbalances and metabolic health.

Research and experience show that addressing metabolic health and hormonal balance can lead to significant improvements in weight management and overall wellness. For instance, studies have indicated that individuals who follow a program focusing on these areas can see a reduction in body fat percentage by up to 15-20% within the first six months. It all starts with optimizing our metabolic health.

Metabolic health refers to our body's ability to efficiently convert food into energy while maintaining optimal blood sugar, cholesterol, and blood pressure levels. Balanced metabolism leads to higher energy, effective weight management, and reduced chronic disease risk. Hormonal imbalances, however, can upset this equilibrium, resulting in weight gain, fatigue, and various health issues.

The R4 System targets these essential health aspects, fostering an environment where your body can restore balance, thrive, and go through a transformation that lasts a lifetime and changes as your preferences do as well. Through evidence-based nutritional guidance, tailored exercise plans, and lifestyle adjustments, we created this system to provide you with true holistic health and optimal well-being.

At AP Elite Health, we have been refining this process over the past 4 years and it has helped over 800 women. We were inspired to create an approach that bridges the gap between medical (doctors), nutrition specialists, and movement specialists. As you probably know, getting to see one doctor often takes forever, and they will likely refer you to someone who is only available months after that as well. When you see someone who gives you the right medication, they don't specialize in nutrition and vice versa. This is where the root cause remains unsolved. Here, we focus on collaboration and support for your overall health outcomes in the long run. This is why we have a strategic partnership with doctors who understand our holistic approach and work hand in hand with us, allowing our clients to have the best of both worlds in a fraction of the time! With this system and our guidance, you get answers and solutions in days, not months or years. Everything you need is all in one place. Now, let's get into how this system has actually helped hundreds.

Real People, Real Results: The R4 Impact

The R4 system is proven, and we have the results to show it. Let's start with the case of Linda, a 48-year-old navigating the complexities of menopause. Linda came to me when she struggled with weight gain, hot flashes, and mood swings, which made her feel at odds with her body. Through the R4 System's Rebalance phase, Linda began to correct her hormonal imbalances, adopting a diet rich in phytoestrogens and participating in stress-reducing activities, per our recommendations. As she moved through the Revitalize and Reshape phases, her symptoms eased, her energy levels surged, and she rediscovered a sense of harmony and confidence in her body. She's just one of the many clients who found the R4 System to be great for menopause and the changes that come with it.

Alongside Linda's journey, we have Alex, a 35-year-old who battled weight fluctuations and fatigue. Through the R4 System, Alex not only shed 30 pounds but also gained energy and confidence, reshaping not just her physique but her entire life perspective.

The R4 System is a comprehensive approach that can solve tons of health problems, whether you're looking to balance your hormones or simply sustain your weight loss!

Chapter 2
Revitalize – Elevating Your Metabolic Health

I n the Revitalize phase, we embark on a critical and often overlooked journey: significantly increasing your metabolic rate through strategic nutritional enhancement. This step is a must and illuminates the path to sustainable health and body composition changes. Herein lies the key to unlocking true metabolic flexibility and setting the foundation for lasting transformation.

Fueling Your Future: The Truth About Calories & Metabolic Optimization

Let's shift to strategically increasing calories and nourishment, a concept that might seem counterintuitive in the traditional weight loss narrative but is essential for metabolic optimization. The goal is to lift your metabolism to new heights, creating a scenario where, in the subsequent Reshape phase, you're not just eating more than before but also witnessing enhanced results.

By intelligently boosting caloric intake, we recalibrate your body's energy use, liberating it from the constraints of a sluggish metabolism. This deliberate nourishment ensures that your body becomes proficient at burning energy, setting the stage for a more dynamic and responsive metabolic state.

The critical mistake I see many encounter in their wellness journey is bypassing the crucial steps of rebalancing and revitalizing. Without addressing these, the body remains in a state of metabolic conservatism, necessitating uncomfortably low caloric intakes for weight loss due to a downregulated metabolism. This unsustainable approach feeds into the vicious cycle of yo-yo dieting, where temporary weight loss is achieved at the cost of long-term sustainability, leading to inevitable weight regain and psychological distress. We're here to prevent that!

The Revitalize phase is designed to liberate you from the notion that starvation or extreme caloric restriction is the only route to weight loss. Through this phase, we address the underlying issue—a downregulated metabolism—by:

Elevating Your Metabolic Rate: By enhancing your metabolic health, we enable drastic changes in body composition to occur at much more comfortable and sustainable caloric levels. This not only makes weight loss more achievable but also enjoyable, as it moves away from restriction and towards nourishment.

Sustainable Transformation: You need a nourished, well-fueled body for sustainable health transformations. One of my favorite parts of my work is when I see how pleasantly surprised people are to learn that eating adequately doesn't impede weight loss but rather supports a healthier, more responsive metabolic system capable of achieving and maintaining your goals without the constant battle against hunger.

This represents a pivotal shift in understanding and approach. By rebalancing and revitalizing your metabolism, we grant you the ultimate food freedom. This freedom allows for significant body composition improvements to be made on a diet that feels satisfying and sustainable, breaking free from the unsustainable cycle of dietary restrictions and setting a new paradigm for health and wellness.

In essence, the Revitalize phase doesn't just adjust your metabolism; it transforms your relationship with food and your body. It equips you with the knowledge and strategies to fuel your body effectively, ensuring that weight loss and health optimization are not just achievable but sustainable and fulfilling. This is the journey to a liberated, revitalized you—where nourishment and health go hand in hand, setting you free from the constraints of past dietary struggles and yo-yo dieting.

Chapter 3
Reshape – The Peak of Transformation

The Reshape phase represents the peak of your transformation within the R4 System. It's a moment many strive to reach, yet few achieve without the foundational work of the preceding phases. This is the stage where the magic happens, where effort is amplified into remarkable results, sculpting a physique that mirrors your dedication and hard work.

Many attempt to jump straight into what they perceive as the "results phase," eager to see immediate changes in their body composition. However, without the crucial groundwork laid in the Rebalance and Revitalize phases, such attempts are often met with frustration and minimal progress. It's like trying to build a house starting from the roof without laying a solid foundation first. The body, much like any well-constructed edifice, requires a base of balanced hormones and a primed metabolism to truly transform.

You, however, are now among the select few who understand the importance of this groundwork. By adhering to the preparatory stages, you've set yourself up for success in the Reshape phase, where your efforts will soon be exponentially rewarded!

The Reshape phase is not merely about working harder; it's about working smarter, leveraging the physiological enhancements achieved through meticulous preparation. Here, we optimize hormonal function to favor lean muscle development and fat loss, something that is only possible with a metabolism that has been carefully calibrated for peak performance.

With your metabolism now in high gear, nutritional adjustments are made to support and sustain muscle growth while continuing to shed fat. This is a fine balance, achieved through precise caloric intake and macronutrient ratios that fuel your workouts and recovery, without compromising the lean gains made.

In the Reshape phase, all your previous efforts starts to manifest in significant, visible changes. This stage is where the full spectrum of transformation unfolds—not just in weight loss but across several dimensions of health and wellness. Here are some specific results you can look forward to:

The targeted strength training and nutritional strategies designed to optimize muscle synthesis come to fruition, revealing a more defined and toned physique. This phase accentuates muscle contours and enhances overall body composition.

As your body becomes more adept at utilizing energy, you may notice an increase in metabolic rate. This doesn't just aid in further weight management but also contributes to a feeling of increased vitality and well-being.

The combination of muscular strength, endurance, and flexibility improvements makes everyday activities easier and enhances performance in sports or physical hobbies. With your body better fueled and more physically fit, one of the most significant changes you'll likely notice is also a sustained boost in energy levels. This increase in energy can positively impact all areas of your life, from work productivity to social interactions.

Physical health and mental well-being are deeply intertwined. As you progress through the Reshape phase, the physical exertion coupled with improved nutrition can lead to better mental clarity, focus, and even mood stabilization. This phase can also lead to improvements in various health markers, including blood pressure, blood sugar levels, and cholesterol profiles, thereby reducing the risk of chronic diseases such as type 2 diabetes, heart disease, and certain forms of cancer.

The exercise regimen in this phase is tailored to maximize efficiency. Strength training takes precedence, structured to enhance muscle hypertrophy and metabolic rate. Yet, it's the quality of these workouts, not just the quantity, that makes the difference, thanks to the resilient foundation you've built.

Celebrating the Peak: When Effort Yields Results

Reaching the Reshape phase is a cause for celebration. It's here that you begin to see the tangible fruits of your labor. Your body responds more readily to your efforts, with each workout and meal moving you closer to your ultimate physique goals. This phase is the embodiment of the phrase "now we're cooking with gas" – your metabolic and hormonal engines are optimized, and you're able to push forward with momentum that was previously unreachable.

The Select Few: Joining the Ranks of True Transformers

By navigating the initial phases of rebalancing and revitalizing, you've earned your place among a select group who truly understand what it takes to experience sustainable transformation after escaping the yo-yo dieting trap. This sets you apart and ensures that you'll never fall into the trap of seeking shortcuts or overlooking the foundational elements of health and fitness.

In the Reshape phase, every effort is amplified, each drop of sweat contributes to a larger tide of change, and your commitment is mirrored in the sculpting of your physique. This is the peak of the mountain, not just a high point on your journey, but a celebration of what it means to achieve through informed, strategic effort.

As you stand at the peak of the Reshape phase, remember that this isn't just about reaching a destination. It's about embracing a process that transforms not only your body but your entire approach to health and fitness. This phase is a testament to the power of preparation, the importance of a solid foundation, and the incredible potential of your body to respond when everything aligns. Welcome to the pinnacle of transformation – where your efforts meet exponential results, and your journey reflects the depth of your dedication.

Chapter 4
Sustaining Your Health Transformation

You've journeyed through the phases of Rebalance, Revitalize, and Reshape, each step bringing you closer to your health and fitness aspirations. Now, you stand at the threshold of the Retain phase, the culmination of your hard work and dedication. This chapter isn't just about maintaining the physical transformations you've achieved; it's about solidifying the lifestyle changes that made those achievements possible. We're here to avoid another unsustainable cycle and step into long-lasting health!

Intuitive Eating: Your Pathway to Food Freedom

The Retain phase heralds a significant shift towards intuitive eating, an approach that champions listening to your body's hunger and fullness cues over adhering to strict dietary rules. You learned about this in our last book, but let's do a little refresh. This method fosters a peaceful relationship with food, where eating becomes an act of self-care, not restriction. By focusing on how foods make you feel, you learn to choose nourishments that satisfy both your body and soul, paving the way for sustainable eating habits. This begins with mindfulness.

A transformation of the body is incomplete without a transformation of the mind. The mindset shifts you've cultivated—embracing progress over perfection, viewing food as nourishment, and recognizing exercise as a celebration of what your body can do—are the bedrock of your new life. This is crucial for navigating life's ups and downs without falling back into old patterns.

Living your transformation means integrating the lessons learned into all aspects of your life. It involves making lifestyle adjustments that support your new, balanced approach to health and fitness. Whether it's prioritizing sleep, managing stress, or fostering relationships that uplift you, these changes are integral to retaining your transformation.

I've seen tons of people thrive in the Retain phase, and I'm sure you'll be next. For instance, people like Maria, who after years of yo-yo dieting, found balance through intuitive eating and a newfound love for yoga, demonstrating that it's possible to maintain a healthy body composition and vibrant health even when life throws curveballs. Or John, who overcame significant stress-related eating habits by adopting stress management techniques, illustrating the power of mindset in sustaining physical transformations.

As you embrace the Retain phase, remember that this is a celebration of a new normal—one where health and confidence are not fleeting goals but stable fixtures in your life. It's not too good to be true! It's a phase that's not about clinging tightly to achievements but about living freely within the sustainable practices you've established. You are now equipped with the tools, knowledge, and mindset to navigate your health journey confidently, no matter what comes your way.

Welcome to the Retain phase, where your transformed body and improved health are just the beginning of a life lived with intention, balance, and joy.

Chapter 5
Beyond the Basics - Specialized Strategies for Lasting Success

Welcome to Chapter 6, where we delve into strategies for those who have navigated the core phases of the R4 Transformation System and are ready to integrate new, sophisticated techniques into their wellness routine. It's about enhancing what works, exploring new horizons, and solidifying your commitment to a lifestyle of vibrant health.

Carb Cycling: Normalizing Your Hormonal Responses

Carb pulsing, also known as carb cycling, is a nutritional strategy that involves varying carbohydrate intake on a daily, weekly, or monthly basis. The goal of carb pulsing is to optimize the body's metabolic and hormonal responses to carbs based on activity levels, goals, and individual metabolic health. By alternating between high-carb and low-carb days, carb pulsing aims to maximize fat loss, enhance muscle growth, improve insulin sensitivity, and prevent metabolic plateaus.

Feasting and Fasting: Optimizing Your Metabolism

Feast and fast strategies involve alternating periods of eating more freely (feasting) with periods of restricted calorie intake or complete fasting (fasting). This approach is designed to harness the metabolic and hormonal benefits of both eating patterns to support weight loss, improve body composition, and enhance overall health.

During feast periods, individuals consume meals that are more calorically dense or larger in volume, often focusing on nutrient-rich foods to maximize nourishment. These periods are usually aligned with workout days or times of higher physical activity to fuel muscle recovery and growth.

Fast periods might range from shorter daily fasts, such as those seen in intermittent fasting protocols like the 16/8 method (16 hours of fasting followed by an 8-hour eating window), to longer 24-hour fasts or days of significantly reduced calorie intake. Fasting periods are utilized to improve insulin sensitivity, promote fat burning, and stimulate autophagy, a process that involves the cleanup of damaged cells, which may contribute to improved health outcomes.

The strategic alternation between feasting and fasting aims to keep the metabolism active and prevent the body from adapting to a single dietary pattern, potentially enhancing the effectiveness of weight management efforts and contributing to greater long-term health benefits.

Intermittent Fasting: Timing for Optimal Health

Intermittent fasting (IF) is a powerful tool for enhancing your health, beyond mere weight management. Its benefits range from improved metabolic health to increased longevity. In fact, a study published in *Cell Metabolism* found that intermittent fasting can decrease insulin resistance, lower blood sugar levels, and improve lipid profiles, all of which are indicators of improved metabolic health!

That being said, the key to successful IF lies in understanding how to integrate it into your life in a way that complements your body's needs and the progress you've made thus far. Don't worry – everything we do is designed to be sustainable. We'll explore different fasting windows, how to align them with your circadian rhythm, and the ways in which IF can boost your metabolic flexibility.

Macro Cycling: How to Master Nutritional Variation

Macro cycling is an advanced approach to nutrition that involves varying your intake of carbohydrates, proteins, and fats to support your body's changing needs—whether you're looking to optimize performance, enhance muscle growth, or accelerate fat loss. This strategy promotes metabolic adaptability and can be particularly effective in breaking through plateaus. We'll guide you through the process of designing a macro cycling plan, taking into account your activity levels, goals, and the insights gained from previous phases.

Cultivating Stress Resilience

Managing stress is not just about avoidance but about building resilience. Let's start by focusing on practical strategies for enhancing your body's resilience to stress, including mindfulness practices, breathwork, and physical activities that reduce cortisol levels. By cultivating stress resilience, you not only safeguard your physical health but also ensure that your mental well-being supports your ongoing transformation journey. Managing stress is the key to lasting change!

Supplements can play a supportive role in achieving and maintaining optimal health, but knowing when and how to incorporate them is crucial. We'll provide a thoughtful overview of supplements that complement the R4 Transformation System, including those that support hormonal balance, digestive health, and nutritional deficiencies. This guidance is about making informed choices that bolster your health without overshadowing the foundational principles of balanced nutrition and lifestyle.

Preventing and Overcoming Plateaus: Strategies for Continued Success

Even with a solid foundation, encountering plateaus is a common part of any health journey. Each advanced technique you integrate should be seen as a tool—not just for enhancing your current success but for building a sustainable, adaptable approach to health and wellness. This is about empowering you to become your own best health advocate, equipped with the knowledge and skills to navigate the complexities of your body's needs through all of life's stages.

Embrace these advanced strategies as part of your ever-evolving health narrative, where lasting success is not just a goal but a way of being.

Chapter 6
The AP Elite Health Community –
Your Support Network

Welcome to Your New Health Family!

Embarking on a health journey can be terrifying, which is why we're here to make it a profound experience that reshapes not just your body, but your entire life. This path isn't meant to be walked alone. At AP Elite Health, we share support, guidance, and ambition. Here, we understand that the strength of one is amplified by the support of many.

Within the AP Elite Health Community, you're never just a number or an anonymous face. You're part of a family that cheers on your victories and supports you through challenges. Our community is built on the foundation of mutual encouragement, where every member's journey is valued and contributes to the collective inspiration of the group.

We're all about accountability. Knowing you have a supportive group awaiting your updates, celebrating your progress, and encouraging you through plateaus can be incredibly motivating. It transforms your personal commitment into a shared endeavor, elevating your sense of responsibility towards your goals.

At the heart of the AP Elite Health Community is our coaching program, designed to offer personalized guidance tailored to your unique journey. Our coaches are not just experts in their fields; they are passionate advocates for your success, dedicated to providing the insights and adjustments needed to navigate your transformation with confidence.

To say that our plans are personalized is an understatement. Beyond generic advice, our coaches dive deep into your individual needs, crafting strategies that address your specific challenges and goals. This personalized approach ensures that your path to health and fitness is as unique as you are.

As part of our community, you gain access to a wealth of knowledge through workshops, seminars, and direct interactions with health and fitness experts. This continuous learning environment keeps you at the forefront of wellness innovation, constantly enriching your journey with new insights.

> *Join the hundreds of other women who are optimizing their health for years to come.*

As you close this book, consider this an invitation not just to change your life but to become part of a movement toward sustained health and vitality. We're more than a support network; it's a launching pad for lifelong transformation and growth. Here, you're not undertaking a temporary diet or fitness regimen but embarking on a journey to reclaim and rediscover your health, with a family of like-minded individuals by your side.

Whether you're seeking motivation, accountability, or personalized guidance, the AP Elite Health Community is ready to welcome you. Together, we can achieve more than any of us could alone. Join us, and let's move forward into a future where your health and happiness are not just hoped for but lived every day.

If you're ready to take your health and fitness to the next level, to be supported, challenged, and celebrated, the AP Elite Health Community awaits. It's time to transform not just your body but your life. And we're here, every step of the way. Welcome to the family.

Glossary

Basal Metabolic Rate (BMR): The number of calories your body needs to perform basic life-sustaining functions, such as breathing, circulation, cell production, and nutrient processing, while at rest.

Caloric Deficit: A state in which you consume fewer calories than your body expends, leading to weight loss.

Circadian Rhythm: The natural, internal process that regulates the sleep-wake cycle and repeats roughly every 24 hours, affecting various bodily functions including hormone release and metabolism.

Hormonal Balance: The equilibrium in the body's hormones, which is crucial for optimal health. Hormones are chemical messengers that impact various functions, from growth and metabolism to mood and reproductive health.

Intermittent Fasting (IF): An eating pattern that cycles between periods of fasting and eating. It does not specify which foods to eat but rather when you should eat them.

Macronutrients: The three main types of nutrients used by the body for energy: carbohydrates, proteins, and fats.

Macro Cycling: The practice of varying the amount of carbohydrates, proteins, and fats consumed on a daily, weekly, or monthly basis to achieve specific health and fitness goals.

Metabolic Flexibility: The body's ability to efficiently switch between burning different types of fuel (such as fats and carbohydrates) based on availability and demand.

Metabolic Health: A spectrum of biochemical and physiological markers that indicate how efficiently the body processes and uses energy. Optimal metabolic health is characterized by balanced blood sugar levels, healthy blood pressure, and appropriate lipid profiles, among other factors.

Mindfulness: The practice of being fully present and engaged in the moment, aware of your thoughts and feelings without distraction or judgment. It is often used as a stress-reduction technique.

Plateau: A period during which there is no significant progress in achieving fitness or weight loss goals, despite continuing with workouts and proper nutrition.

Supplements: Products taken orally that contain one or more ingredients (like vitamins or amino acids) intended to supplement one's diet and are not considered food.

Sustainable Eating: A dietary approach that focuses on consuming foods that are healthful to the environment and the body. It often involves eating locally grown, organic foods and reducing consumption of processed and packaged foods.

Workout Intensity: The level of effort or exertion that an individual applies in physical exercise, often measured by the heart rate, sweat rate, and perceived exertion.

This glossary is designed to enrich your understanding of key concepts and terms used throughout this book, supporting your journey through the R4 Transformation System and towards lasting health and freedom.

Disclaimer

This book and its content are provided for informational purposes only and are not intended as medical advice, diagnosis, or treatment. The information contained herein is not meant to replace professional medical advice or to apply to individuals with specific medical conditions. Before beginning any new diet or exercise program, including any aspects of the R4 Transformation System outlined in this book, it is recommended that you consult with a qualified healthcare professional to ensure that it is appropriate for your individual circumstances and health needs.

The authors, contributors, and publisher of this book disclaim any liability or loss, personal or otherwise, resulting from the procedures and information contained herein. No guarantee can be made regarding the outcomes of following the advice provided in this book. The statements made about health, nutrition, fitness, and wellness have not been evaluated by the Food and Drug Administration or any other regulatory body and are not intended to diagnose, treat, cure, or prevent any disease.

AP Elite Health and its representatives do not assume any responsibility for errors, omissions, or contrary interpretations of the subject matter herein. Participation in any dietary or exercise program described in this book is at the sole choice and risk of the reader.

As health and nutrition research continuously evolves, we do not guarantee the accuracy, completeness, or timeliness of any information presented in this book. The use of this book does not create a doctor-patient relationship between you and the authors or publisher.

By using this book, you agree to the terms of this disclaimer. If you do not agree with these terms, you are not authorized to use or access the information provided.

www.ingramcontent.com/pod-product-compliance
Lightning Source LLC
Chambersburg PA
CBHW051902250726

48659CB00006B/2361